Table of Contents

Introduction

When you look at the mirror, you already know how confident you are and how it brings you to move forward with your day. Healthy skin matters most in our everyday undertakings. Consciously and even unconsciously, it affects our decisions in life even to the smallest details in our actions like how are we going to stand up with the crowd having the confidence to walk and brag about what we've got.

Not only does this boost our confidence towards people but also it expresses the sign of having a healthy body, glowing from the inside which makes bacteria run out for homage!

But here is the problem that we usually overlook. One is when we are too inattentive enough to jeopardize our skin health through bad eating habit. The law of consequence is always correct that when you eat healthy you will be healthy otherwise you will suffer seeing a clumsy, pale, unhealthy person when you stand in front of the mirror!

What problems do we face when our body reacts in a different way like it can't face a day without red alerts- and in a worst case, when our body protector, the skin, has the problem itself because instead of its role to block foreign, uninvited guests from entering our body, it has already become colonized because of its few fighting agent and weak prevention system?

Do you want this condition be your reputation for good? Definitely, you will not bet this forever into your life. Everybody does not want this. Everybody has to get rid of this or face this. Maybe, it's a part of one of the most challenging areas in our lives where we need to be "upgraded" as we aged.

But how do we face this problem when the problem is within ourselves? Yes. The start depends on us. The changes begin in us. Decision to change the way we deal with our body, the way we feed nutrients to our skin, the way we choose a set of pattern in our lifestyle is a big step to removing our old skin and becoming a new us!

However, in most cases, such decision has become just a prisoner of our own fantasies. Words are easy to explain, and in reality, they are way hard to follow. Or even if you have followed, the consistency takes the question mark for the main point of this sentence, how are you going to maintain such decision every day? Do you think you can just get rid of the temptation to eat your favorite companions in eating that easy? Absolutely, you can't just jump off the base of the mountain right at the top without undergoing extreme climbing all the way. You can't let a new-born baby grow into an adult in just a matter of a second or a seed to become a tree with just a flip of the page in this book!

Yes, everything has a step including your decision to change the way you are now to achieve such dream in you in becoming healthy, glowing, beautiful you. But the few first steps are difficult to take yet because in those stages you are saying goodbye to the old you promising not to ever come back. It will be pretty useless to do a hard work for yourself when you just turn around and go back to who you were before. However, in the long run, you will then taste the worth of your sacrifices to peel off your old self and discover something beautiful inside.

This book will help you achieve your dream. If you only follow what this says with no doubt, no what ifs, no back thoughts, you will release the fantasies inside of you and see them realized. I suggest you to have a firm decision of this beginning journey towards becoming a beautiful healthy, glowing you!

Chapter 1 :Bad Eating Habits Hamper Your Skin

Apparently, those foods that flirt with our mouth are those that can be very bad for our health. Bad eating habits definitely eat our health away and it can damage our skin too.

Healthy skin is an indicator of a healthy lifestyle. Unfortunately the modern day diet consists a lot of stuff which are bad for you-greasy fries, chips, soda and the list goes endless. Not only these foods alone can cause an aging, ghoulish, but eating them can lead to obesity, heart diseases, bad mood and even cloudy thinking.

Some ruining habits to your skin are frequent snacking and skipping breakfast, stress and mindless eating. Frequent snacking will lead you to eating junk foods, sweets or sodium-rich foods oftentimes in which unconsciously you have no control of. Skipping breakfast makes your skin dry. When you wake up in the morning, your skin cells had just recovered from your all-day work and as your body needs energy at the start of the day and so does your skin. Mindless eating jeopardizes every skin care you have no matter how mindful you are at it. What you take inside your body affects more than what you apply on your skin. Thus, it is more important to eat healthy foods than apply even expensive skin care products.

Such involuntary patterns can invade of what is supposed to be a healthy, resistant skin. On the other way around, these can cause a weak resistance against skin infection, early signs of aging, dry and rough skin and most especially bad signs and symptoms of your general health.

Overall, no matter how you put care to your outside appearance, what you do inside has greater effects. Hence, it is rather more important to start from within!

Symptoms of Bad Skin and How to Fix it with Good Food

Signs and symptoms of your skin problems bring a message about a similar condition. However these two possess different meanings. Signs are things that other people see but what you see in you is otherwise called symptoms.

Symptoms can help you trace your own skin problem thus you will immediately proceed to potential solutions before other people can figure it out. Some symptoms that you have bad skin (can also be called a sign) is when you notice you are always prone to acne anywhere in your body including your face. These can be resolved when you take a bath regularly because acne is dirt that actually clogs your skin pores making bacteria dwell in it. But it doesn't tell the whole problem. In most cases, these are caused by the foods you take! Caffeinated beverages, sugar and carbohydrate-rich foods, dairy products can trigger for acne to grow. Health conscious always suggest consume only fresh foods like protein-rich, vegetables, healthy fats from fish and eggs.

The acne-prone skin is just one of the bad skin signs and symptoms. There is a lot of it that you can experience and of course one symptom is that you don't feel good about your looks. Such problem can be solved when you stick to a healthy and balanced diet.

Fruits and vegetables are always nature's best choice. You may never have these all the time but there are refined products that contain of it like yogurt, cocoa powder (help hydrate your skin), soy milk and green tea.

In spite of all the good foods that are suggested by this book. You shall never forget a bland-tasting nature's health soldier against all skin odds—water. Water can help you a lot in cleansing your body and skin inside and out. Plus, it is down-to-earth available all the time!

Smoking Effect to Skin

Smoking is popularly known as the major enemy of everyone's health. There are a number of cases that are linked to this such as lung cancer and heart diseases. This act of smoke inhalation from tobaccos or any other sources can tremendously ruin not only your internal organ or other functioning system but also your skin! Smoking can definitely increase the rate of aging- known otherwise as premature aging.

Premature aging is an early sign of aging. Hence, it takes place not in the time appropriate for this. Smoking looses your skin elasticity, dries your skin due to its absorbent capacity of Vitamin A and moisture from your body.

Smoking can also narrow your blood vessels. As a result, oxygen can hardly reach to your blood cells leading to a very delay healing of your skin cuts and wounds.

Another worst case that smoking can do to your skin is skin cancer. You see people who are smokers that tend to be older in their looks but younger in their age. You also see others whose wounds have seemingly stayed on their skin for a quite longer time. However, in other cases you see people that have gross look blood clot and puss somewhere on different skin areas such as ears, lips, faces, legs, toes or even tongues! These wound-looking things on their skin are not mere wounds but are skin cancers!

Skin cancers due to smoking are very dangerous and can never be healed most of the time. This is because as you absorb smoke in your body, it not only affects your breathing organ but it also slows down all functioning systems of your body including your blood flows, oxygen intake of your blood cells and your immune system.

The law of consequence will never be defied. Once you do a thing, you will always have to face its nature's just offense! So, quit smoking today or not, avoid the curiosity of exploring it or not, begin a healthy lifestyle or ignore, your choice will always be your life!

Chapter 2. : Recipes

Breakfast

Strawberry and Banana Smoothie

Preparation time: 5 min.

Cooking time: 3 min.

Servings: 3-4

Ingredients

- 150 ml characteristic yogurt
- 250 g strawberries, hulled
- 1 ripe banana
- 15 ml spoon clear nectar
- 300 ml low-fat milk

Directions

1. Peel the banana and cut into small chunks.
2. Throw all the ingredients into a food processor one by one.
3. Blend until smooth and serve fresh.

Green Waffle

Preparation time: 10

Cooking time: 20

Servings: 5-6

Ingredients

- 4 eggs
- 1/2 tsp preparing powder
- ½ tbsp vanilla extract
- 1 tbsp coconut flour
- 1 tbsp honey
- 1 tbsp Cinnamon

Directions

1. Preheat the waffle maker.
2. In a bowl whisk the eggs with vanilla extract.
3. Add the cinnamon, honey, coconut flour and preparing powder to it.
4. Stir well and make a smooth batter.
5. Pour into the waffle maker and heat up.
6. Repeat in batches and serve immediately.

Fig bircher muesli

Preparation Time: 10 minutes

Servings: 6

Ingredients:

- 2 1/2cups natural muesli
- 1 1/2 cups apple juice
- 1 cup reduced-fat plain yogurt
- 3/4 cup chopped dried figs
- 3 fresh figs, quartered
- 3/4 cup reduced-fat milk
- 2 tbsp raw honey
- 1/4 cup slivered almonds, toasted

Directions

1. Combine the yogurts, honey, dried figs, muesli and apple juice into a bowl.
2. Give it a good stir.
3. Fridge overnight and garnish with nuts before serving.

Fruit skewers

Preparation Time: 10 minutes

Cooking Time: 5 minutes

Servings: 6

Ingredients:

- 1 rock melon, peeled
- 1 1/2 cups white sugar
- 1 honeydew melon, peeled
- 800g pineapple, peeled
- 1 orange, rind shredded, juiced
- 1 cup water
- 1 vanilla bean, halved lengthways

Directions

1. Cut all the fruits into 2 inch cubes.
2. It is important that the fruits are of equal size.
3. Thread the fruits into metal skewers.
4. Fridge for about an hour.
5. In a pan heat up the water with sugar.
6. Add orange juice, orange rind, and vanilla to it.
7. Bring this to a boil and take off the heat.
8. Let it cool and afterwards drizzle on top of the skewers.

Sparkling Fruit Salad

Preparation Time: 1 hour

Servings: 6

Ingredients:

- 1/2 pineapple
- 1 cup pink sparkling wine, chilled
- 2 tbsp mint, chopped
- 2 1/2 tbsp pure icing sugar
- 1/4 honeydew melon
- 1/4 rock melon
- 500g seedless watermelon

Directions

1. Peel the pineapple, honeydew melon and seedless watermelon.
2. Cut them into semi thin slices.
3. In a serving bowl, layer the fruits so it looks visually stimulating.
4. Combine the wine with the sugar.
5. Stir well to dissolve the sugar and pour over the fruits.
6. Fridge for an hour and serve.

Low Carb Pancake Crepes

Preparation Time: 10 minutes

Cooking Time: 10 minutes

Servings: 2

Ingredients:

1 tsp of almond butter

2 eggs, beaten

1 tsp of cinnamon

3 oz cream cheese, softened

1 tbsp of sugar-free syrup

Directions

1. Combine the cream cheese with the eggs.
2. Sprinkle the cinnamon to it.
3. Pour the syrup in and mix well.
4. Make sure there are no lumps.
5. In a pan melt the butter and pour the batter in batches using a ladle.
6. Golden fry them on each side and serve immediately.

Blueberry pancakes

Preparation Time: 10 minutes

Cooking Time: 10 minutes

Servings: 2

Ingredients:

20g almond butter

375g pancake mix

2 cups frozen blueberries

1/2 cup icing sugar

1 lemon, zest and juice

3 eggs, beaten

1 cup water

1/2 cup yogurt, to serve

Directions

1. In a non-stick pan toss the icing sugar with lemon zest.
2. Add the blueberries to it.
3. Toss for about 5-6 minutes and then take off the heat.
4. Let the mixture cool and them add the eggs.
5. Add the water to it and create a smooth batter.
6. In a non-stick pan melt the butter and fry the pancakes golden brown.
7. Serve immediately with yogurt.

Date Pancakes

Preparation Time: 10 minutes

Cooking Time: 10 minutes

Servings: 4

Ingredients:

1 tbsp of almond butter

½ cup of date paste

2 tbsp of raw honey

A pinch of cardamom

3 eggs

½ cup of almond flour

A pinch of cinnamon

1 cup of almond milk

A pinch of sea salt

Direction

1. In a bowl combine the flour with milk.
2. Whisk in the eggs and mix well.
3. Add the honey, salt and cinnamon to it and make the mix smooth.
4. Now melt the butter in a non-stick pan and fry the pancakes golden brown in batches.

Delicious yogurt smoothie

Preparation time: 10 min
Servings: 2

Ingredients:

1 banana

½ cup of fresh almond yogurt

Fresh mint

Ice cubes

1 tbsp of raw honey

A pinch of cinnamon

Water if needed

Directions:

Start off by peeling the banana and chop it up thinly.

1. Throw the banana with yogurt into a blender.
2. Add some water to it if needed.
3. Blend for about 3 minutes.
4. Add the ice cubes, mint, honey and cinnamon and blend for another minute.
5. Serve immediately.

Mango Smoothie

Preparation time: 10 min
Servings: 2

Ingredient:

A pinch of cinnamon

1 mango

Ice cubes
Fresh mint

1 ½ cup of soy milk

A pinch of sea salt

Directions:
Start by peeling the mango and get rid of the cord.

1. Cut it into small pieces.
2. Throw the mango with the milk into a blender.
3. Add the mint, ice cubes, cinnamon and salt to it.
4. Blend for about 5 minutes or until the mix is smooth.
5. Serve fresh.

Lunch

Paleo Sushi with Salmon & Avocado

Preparation time: 30 min
Cooking time: 5 min

Servings: 2-4

Ingredients:

- 1 salmon steak
- 2 cucumbers
- ½ onion, diced
- 1 tbsp olive oil
- Paprika to taste
- Salt and pepper to taste
- 1 avocado
- Tamari

Directions:

1. Season the salmon with salt, pepper, paprika.
2. In a nonstick pan heat the oil.
3. Fry the salmon for about 2 minutes on each side.
4. Transfer into a plate and let it cool.
5. Get rid of all the bones.
6. Combine the salmon with onion.
7. Take the cucumbers and peel them.
8. Cut thick circles out of the cucumber and get rid of the seeds.
9. Now you would have cucumber rings.
10. Fill half of it with the salmon mix and the rest of it with avocado.

11. Repeat it with the rest and serve immediately.

Caesar Salad Spears

Preparation time: 20 min
Cooking time: 10 min

Servings: 4

Ingredients:

- 1/4 cup extra-virgin olive oil
- 7 Belgian endives
- 1/4 cup mayonnaise
- 1/2 tsp finely grated lemon zest
- 3 anchovy fillets, mashed
- 1/4 tsp salt
- Pepper to taste
- 2 tbsp fresh lemon juice
- 2 cups diced white bread
- 1/4 cup cheese
- 1 small garlic clove, smashed

Directions:

1. Preheat your oven on 350°F.
2. Mix the bread with 2 tbsp of olive oil. Add salt and pepper.
3. Now place that over baking dish and bake for only 10 minutes.
4. In that same bowl, mash those anchovies, add the garlic. Season with salt.
5. Pour in mayo, the lemon zest and the lemon juice. Mix it with the mash anchovies mixture.
6. Throw in the rest of the olive oil. Throw in the 1/4 cup of cheese.

7. In a bowl, throw in the endives, pour in the mixtures on top and finally the cheese.

8. Toss around and serve immediately.

Braised Lamb

Preparation time: 15 min

Cooking time: 2 hours

Yield: Serves 4.

Ingredients

- 1 1/4 cup stock
- 3 potatoes, cut into chunks
- 2 Lamb shanks
- 1 onion, chopped
- 2 tbsp olive oil
- 2 celery stalks, chopped
- Salt
- 2 carrots, chopped
- 1 garlic clove, minced
- 1 tsp dried oregano
- 2 tsp fresh thyme
- 1 tsp fresh rosemary, chopped,
- 1 bay leaf
- 1/2 cup of fresh mint leaves
- 3/4 cup raisins, soaked in sherry for hours

Directions:

1. Start by preheating the oven to 350° F.
2. Season the lamb shanks using salt and pepper.
3. In a pan heat the olive oil and fry the lamb for about 5 minutes.
4. Stir in the onion, celery, carrot and toss around for 5 minutes.
5. Stir in the potatoes and toss for about 5 minutes.
6. Stir in the garlic, herbs, raisins and toss.

7. Pour in the mixture into a boil and then pour the stock.
8. Simmer the mixture for 10 minutes.
9. Pour in onto a baking dish and bake for about 2 hours on the preheated oven.
10. Serve hot.

Healthy Paleo Crock Pot Tuna

Preparation time: 20 min
Cooking time: 3 hour

Servings: 4

Ingredients:

14 Oz Tuna

1/3 cup vegetable broth

Paleo friendly Cream of celery soup

3 tbsp Paleo bread crumbs

10 Oz green pea sods

1 tbsp olive oil

2 tbsp dried parsley flakes

10 Oz cooked zucchini noodles

2/3 cup coconut milk

Directions:

1. In a crock pot grease some oil.
2. Combine the vegetable broth with milk, tuna, soup, parsley, green pea sods.
3. Give it a good stir.
4. Stir in the zucchini noodles.
5. Stir in the bread crumbs and whisk well.
6. Cover with lid and cook for about 3 hours.
7. Serve hot.

Vegetable Quinoa Pilaf

Preparation time: 20 min
Cooking time: 40 min

Servings: 4-6

Ingredients:

2 cups quinoa

1/3 cup lemon juice

4 green onions, thinly sliced

2 zucchini, chopped

4 cups vegetable stock

2 red capsicums, chopped

Olive oil cooking spray

1 eggplant, chopped

2 tbsp fresh oregano leaves

Fresh oregano leaves, to serve

Directions:

1. In a pan pour the broth with the quinoa.
2. Bring the mixture to a boil.
3. Turn the heat to low and simmer for about 10 minutes.
4. Stir occasionally. Check if the quinoa is tender and then turn the heat off.
5. Cover with lid and let it rest for 10 minutes.
6. In a pan spray the oil and stir in eggplant, capsicum and toss for 2 minutes.
7. Toss for 10 minutes and stir in the zucchini, oregano and onions.
8. Toss for another 10 minutes.
9. Pour this to the quinoa and add in the lemon juice.
10. Serve with pepper and oregano on top.

Barbecued Corn with Tomato and Almond Salad

Preparation time: 10 min
Cooking time: 10 min

Servings: 4

Ingredients:

4 fresh corn cobs, husks removed

200g cherry tomatoes

1 tbsp red wine vinegar

1 shallot

1/2 cup basil leaves

2 tbsp olive oil

Salt and pepper to taste

1/4 cup flaked almonds, toasted

Directions:

1. Quarter the cherry tomatoes.
2. Cut the shallots into thin pieces.
3. Combine the cherry tomatoes with shallots, oil, and vinegar.
4. Season with salt and pepper to it.
5. Place it into the fridge.
6. Before serving take out of the fridge.
7. Stir in the toasted almonds and the basil to it and stir well.
8. Quarter the corn cobs and drizzle some oil to it.
9. Season it with salt and pepper.
10. Grill the corn for about 5 minutes on each side.
11. Serve with the almond salad.

Carrot and Radish Salad

Preparation time: 10 min
Servings: 4

Ingredients:

- 1 cup fresh mint leaves, torn
- 60ml olive oil
- 1 bunch radish
- 3 carrots
- 60ml fresh lemon juice
- 1 tsp ground cumin
- 1/4 tsp ground cinnamon
- 1 tbsp honey
- 1/4 tsp rosewater essence
- 1 tsp mild paprika
- 2 garlic cloves, finely chopped

Directions:

1. Peel the carrots and cut into thin slices.
2. Combine the lemon juice with honey, add in the oil, garlic, rosewater essence, paprika, cumin and cinnamon into a bowl.
3. Season with salt and pepper.
4. In a separate combine the radish with carrots.
5. Stir in the mint leaves.
6. Drizzle the lemon juice mix to it and coat well.
7. Serve fresh.

Yummy Ratatouille

Preparation time: 15 min
Cooking time: 25 min

Servings: 4

Ingredients:

- 3 tomatoes, chopped
- 2 zucchini
- 1 tbsp olive oil
- 3 tbsp vinegar
- 1 eggplant
- 2 red capsicums, thinly sliced
- 2 garlic cloves, crushed
- 1 tbsp red wine vinegar

Directions:

1. Mince the eggplant and cut the zucchini into thin slices.
2. In a pan heat the oil and fry the capsicum with the garlic for about 4 minutes.
3. Stir in the eggplants and toss for 3 minutes.
4. Add in the zucchini and toss for another 3 minutes.
5. Add in the tomatoes and the vinegar.
6. Toss for about 10 minutes.
7. Add some water if needed.
8. Season with salt and pepper and toss for 5 minutes.
9. Keep tossing until the sauce is thick.
10. Serve hot.

Dinner

Lamb Stew

Preparation time: 20 min
Cooking time: 1 hour

Servings: 4

Ingredients

3 lamb shoulder

1 cup dry red wine

1 onion, peeled and chopped

6 cloves garlic, crushed and peeled

1 cup chicken stock

2 tsp sweet paprika

1 roasted red bell peppers

1 ripe tomato

1/2 cup dry white wine

1 sprig rosemary, chopped

1 bay leaf

2 tbsp parsley

2 tbsp extra-virgin olive oil

Salt

Freshly ground black pepper

Directions

1. Cut the red bell pepper into thin strips.
2. Peel the tomato and deseed it. Chop it.
3. Marinade the lamb with the garlic, white wine, and the rosemary.
4. Fridge it for about 3 hours.
5. In a pan heat the oil and fry the lamb brown for about 10 minutes on each side.

6. Take off the heat and meat as it browns.
7. Fry the onions into the same pan for 5 minutes.
8. Add the remaining garlic and season with paprika.
9. Add the roasted peppers, bay leaf, parsley and the tomatoes.
10. Toss around for 2 minutes and then pour the wine.
11. Bring the mixture to a boil and turn the heat to medium low.
12. Simmer for about 15-20 minutes.
13. Finally pour in the chicken stock and again bring it to boil.
14. Simmer for another 2 hours.
15. Season with salt and pepper and serve hot.

Crock Pot Fish with Orange

Preparation time: 20 min
Cooking time: 1 hour

Servings: 3-4

Ingredients:

1 ½ pounds White fish fillets

2 tsp grated lemon rind

½ cup chopped onions

2 tsp grated orange rind

1 tbsp Vegetable oil

Parsley sprigs

5 tbsp chopped parsley

Salt

Pepper

Directions:

1. Season with fish fillets with salt and pepper.
2. Marinade it with orange rind, parsley, onions, vegetable oil and lemon rind.
3. Place into a crockpot and cover with the lid.
4. Cook on low flame for about 1 hour.
5. Serve hot.

Crock Pot Catfish Chowder

Preparation time: 20 min
Cooking time: 1.5 hours

Servings: 4

Ingredients:

12 Oz evaporated coconut milk

2 pounds Catfish fillets

2 cups Water

½ tsp Pepper

4 potatoes

Salt to taste

1 onion, chopped

1tbsp olive oil

Directions:

1. Peel the potatoes and cut it into bite size chunks.
2. In a pan heat half the oil and fry the onion for about 2 minutes.
3. Place the rest of the oil into a crock pot.
4. Add the fried onion, with the fish fillets.
5. Stir in the potatoes, coconut milk, water, salt and pepper.
6. Cover with the lid and cook on low flame for about 1.5 hours.
7. Serve hot.

Homemade Paleo Bone Broth

Preparation time: 10 min
Cooking time: 20 min

Servings: 4

Ingredients:

- 4 pounds of beef knuckle bones
- 2 pounds of neck bones
- 4 quart of cold water
- 3 large onions, chopped
- 4 celery sticks, chopped
- ¼ cup of vinegar
- 1 tsp of sea salt

Directions:

1. Take a baking sheet and place knuckle bones on it, bake for about 30 minutes on 350F.
2. Now take the neck bones into a crockpot.
3. Add water and vinegar to it and cook on low heat.
4. Once the knuckle bones are browned in the oven, take them off.
5. Add the knuckle bones to the pot.
6. Bring this mixture to a boil on a high heat.
7. Now reduce your heat and simmer the mixture for 12 hours or so.

Baby Brussels Sprouts Slaw

Preparation time: 20 min
Servings: 4

Ingredients:

- 500g baby brussels sprouts
- 75g light sour cream
- 1 tbsp water
- 2 tsp Dijon mustard
- 1 tbsp apple cider vinegar
- 55g hazelnuts, dry-roasted, chopped

Directions:

1. Half the Brussels sprouts.
2. In a bowl combine the sour cream with the Dijon mustard, water and apple cider vinegar.
3. Whisk well and plate up with the Brussels sprouts, sprinkle the hazelnut.
4. Add the sour cream on top.
5. Adjust the seasoning and serve.

Zucchini corn carrot Stew

Preparation time: 10 min
Cooking time: 30 min

Servings: 4

Ingredients:

- 4 cup of vegetable broth
- 1 tbsp of oil
- ½ cup of chopped baby corn
- 1 tsp of paprika
- 1 tsp of cumin
- 2 yellow zucchini, diced
- 1 tsp of turmeric
- 3 carrots, diced
- 2 Green chilies
- 1 tsp of salt

Directions:

1. In a nonstick pan heat the oil.
2. Stir in the onions and toss for about 2 minutes or until it starts to lose its color.
3. Add the carrots, zucchini, baby corn into the pan and toss for about 8 minutes.
4. Add in the chilies, cumin paprika and turmeric and toss for 2 minutes.
5. Pour in the vegetable broth.
6. Cover using a lid and cook for about 30 minutes and serve hot.

Juicy Crab in Lettuce

Preparation time: 10 min
Cooking time: 10 min

Servings: 6

Ingredients:

- 1 cup of cashew nuts
- 1 cup of crab
- ½ cup of chopped spring onions
- ½ tsp of nutmeg
- 2 tbsp of honey
- ½ sp of black pepper
- 1 tbsp of lime juice
- ½ tsp of cumin powder
- Sea salt to taste
- 2 tbsp of olive oil
- A handful of lettuce

Directions:

1. In a nonstick pan heat the olive oil.
2. Stir in the onions and toss for a minute.
3. Stir in the crab and season using salt and pepper.
4. Sprinkle the nutmeg, and cumin.
5. Toss for a minute and take off the heat.
6. In a plain surface place the lettuce.
7. Add the crab filling in the middle and roll it up tightly.
8. Sprinkle with nuts and drizzle with lime juice and honey.

Mushroom soup

Preparation time: 15 min
Cooking time: 1.5 hours

Servings: 6

Ingredients:

1 cup of white mushroom

6 cup vegetable broth

1 cabbage

1 carrot

Salt and pepper to taste

½ cup of cashew paste

Fresh mint, chopped

4 green chilies

1 tsp of ginger garlic paste

2 tbsp of olive oil

Directions:

1. Shred the cabbage into thin pieces.
2. Shred the carrots thinly.
3. In a pressure cooker heat the oil.
4. Fry the cabbage and carrots for about 5 minutes.
5. Stir in the mushroom and toss for 4 minutes.
6. Add the rest of ingredients to it and give it a good stir.
7. Cover and cook on low flame for about 1 hour.
8. Serve hot.

Caramel Apples

Preparation Time: 2 hours

Cooking Time: 25 min

Servings: 4

Ingredients:

- 4 apples
- 1 ¼ cup raw honey
- A Dash of salt
- 1 cup coconut cream

Directions:

1. In a pan pour the coconut cream with honey.
2. Sprinkle the salt to it and turn the heat to medium low.
3. Heat for 20 minutes and then your mix would bubble.
4. Take off the heat and let it cool a little bit.
5. Thread the apples in sticks and then dip the apples into the mix.
6. Place them into a tray and fridge for about 2 hours.
7. Serve cold or room temperature.

Almond with Rosewater Syrup Treat

Preparation Time: 4 hours

Cooking Time: 30 min

Servings: 2

Ingredients:

- 300ml pure coconut cream
- 150g slivered toasted almonds
- 300ml coconut milk
- 1/2 cup raw honey
- 1 1/2 tsp cardamom seeds
- 1/2 tsp rosewater

Directions:

1. Chop the almonds roughly and set aside for now.
2. Combine the coconut milk with the cream and cardamom.
3. Pour that into a large pan.
4. Bring it to a boil and then simmer for 10 minutes.
5. Let it cool down.
6. Once it has cooled down, beat for 10 minutes.
7. Stir in the almonds.
8. Pour into ice cream cups and fridge for 4 hours or overnight.
9. Serve cold.

Apricot and Pistachio Kulfi

Preparation Time: 8 hours

Cooking Time: 20 min

Servings: 2

Ingredients:

- 40g chopped pistachio kernels
- Vegetable oil, to grease
- 10 cardamom pods, bruised
- 375ml coconut milk
- 55g chopped dried apricots

Directions:

1. In a skillet pour the milk.
2. Add the cardamom pods and cook for about 2 min.
3. Turn off the stove and let it cool.
4. Strain once it has cooled off.
5. Stir in the pistachios and apricots and fridge for 8 hours.
6. Serve with mint on top.

Cabbage Pudding

Preparation Time: 1 hour

Cooking Time: 30 minutes

Servings: 4

Ingredients:

- 2 cup of coconut milk
- ½ cup of sucralose
- A pinch of cardamom
- 1 cabbage
- 1 tbsp almond butter
- A pinch of cinnamon

Directions:

1. Shred the cabbage.
2. In a skillet melt the almond butter.
3. Pour in the coconut milk.
4. Sprinkle the cinnamon and cardamom to it.
5. Bring it to a boil and keep stirring.
6. Simmer for about 10 minutes.
7. Add in the sucralose and stir for 5 minutes.
8. Fridge for 1 hour or so and serve cold.

Indian carrot pudding

Preparation time: 20 min
Cooking time: 1 hour

Servings: 4-6

Ingredients:

- 2 cup coconut milk
- 10 green cardamom pods
- 200g of chopped carrots
- 1 tsp vanilla extract
- 1 cinnamon quill
- 50g unsalted almond butter
- 80g sultanas
- 1 tsp finely grated lemon rind
- 6 tbsp of raw honey

Directions:

1. Start by preheating the oven to 350F.
2. Combine the carrots, cinnamon, lemon, milk, butter, cardamom, honey and sultanas into a bowl.
3. Stir well and create a smooth mixture.
4. Pour that into greased round baking dish.
5. Place it onto a tray and pour some water on it.
6. Bake for nearly 40 minutes and then let it cool.
7. Serve cold.

Pumpkin Pudding

Preparation Time: 5 minutes

Cooking Time: 1 minute

Servings: 4

Ingredients:

- 750g pumpkin, peeled, deseeded
- 1/2 cup grated tasty cheese
- 3 eggs, separated
- 1/4 tsp ground nutmeg
- 1/2 cup almond milk

Directions:

1. Preheat the oven to 425F.
2. Cut the pumpkin into small chunks.
3. Boil the pumpkin with water for about 20-30 minutes.
4. Drain well and place into a pan.
5. Mash them using a wooden spoon.
6. In a mixing bowl combine the cheese with egg yolks, milk, salt, nutmeg and pepper.
7. Stir in the mashed pumpkin mix to it and stir well.
8. In another bowl beat the egg whites for about 4 minutes or until fluffy.

9. Pour into a baking dish and place that onto a tray with water.

10. Bake for about 40 minutes.

Papaya Treats

Preparation time: 10 min
Cooking time: 30 min

Servings: 4

Ingredients:

- 1 raw papaya
- ½ cup of coconut milk
- 6 tbsp of raw honey
- 2 tbsp of almond butter
- 1 cardamom
- 1 bay leaf
- 1 cinnamon stick

Directions:

1. Melt the almond butter and fry the papaya for about 8 minutes.
2. Stir in the bay leaf, cinnamon and cardamom and toss for a minute.
3. Add the milk to it and bring it to a boil.
4. Keep stirring occasionally.
5. Make it thickened and then take off the heat.
6. Let it rest for 10 minutes and then create little balls out of them.
7. Serve cold or in room temperature.

Apple Pie Muffins

Preparation Time: 25 minutes

Cooking Time: 35 minutes

Servings: 2

Ingredients:

- ½ cup flour
- ½ tsp salt
- ½ tsp baking soda
- ½ tsp baking powder
- 5 fresh eggs
- 2 egg whites
- 1 large banana (mashed)
- ½ cup almond butter
- 1 tsp vanilla
- 1½ tsp cinnamon
- 1 green apple (chopped)

Directions:

1. Combine all the ingredients except the green chopped apple in a large mixing bowl and stir.
2. Beat the mixture in an electric mixer for about 3 minutes, until it becomes nice and fluffy.
3. Fold in the green apples.
4. Put the mixture in a muffin pan.
5. Bake for at 350 degrees for about 20 minutes. Let it cool before removing the muffins from the pan.

Sweet Potato Muffins

Preparation Time: 25 minutes

Cooking Time: 35 minutes

Servings: 2

Ingredients:

- 1/2 Cup Coconut Flour
- 6 fresh ggs
- 1 1/2 tsp vanilla
- 1 tsp Salt
- 1 tsp Baking Soda
- 2 tsp Cinnamon
- 1/2 c Ground Flax
- 2 Sweet Potatoes or Yams, baked and mashed (remove skins)
- 1 Cup cashew nuts (optional)

Directions:

1. **In a large bowl, whisk together all the dry ingredients you have. Beat the eggs and add dry mixture by spoonfuls until well blended.**
2. **Add the mashed sweet potatoes.**
3. Spoon the batter into the muffin buttered cups. Bake at 350 degrees for around 30-35 minutes.

Skin Care Tips

To start with a healthy lifestyle, one has to figure out the best way on how to start. Your decision to start another life is one great step to a succeeding success of your journey towards your goal-- looking good, feeling good and being good!

I suggest you to have these following steps to start your day off to a new, beautiful and healthy you!

Know your skin type!

Different kinds of skin need different kinds of treatment, you should know yours! There are 5 main types: normal, oily, dry, sensitive and combination.

2. Drink a lot of water.

Drinking water is the most affordable, available of all time to help you provide your skin a fresher and cleaner look inside and outside. Of course, it's no magic that you can instantly get the benefit of it. But as you go along the way, it will become magic! You can definitely see a great effect to your skin after a four-week routine of drinking water 8 glasses a day!

4. Avoid prolonged sun exposure.

Sun's heat can dry your skin. Observe a soil that has been exposed to the sun for a longer time. You'll see cracked areas because water has been dried out! It is the same thing that sun can do to your skin. The cracked soil is similar to your skin wrinkles. When you run out of skin moisture, you'll get a lot of fine lines until it becomes more obvious to look at. I suggest you to always apply sunscreen whenever you go out.

5. Eat fresh foods preferably fruits and vegetables.

Fruits and veggies have natural content of antioxidant that helps renew your skin cells and produce more collagen. They are also rich in other vitamins and minerals that are necessary not only to your skin but also to your overall body health.

These three steps are simple. But there is no simplicity when it comes to their effect on our skin-- somewhat like it's a gift of nature that to change our lifestyle is no hard way. We just have to shift our outlook and here it goes. You will find in every corner of the street of what is important to be fully healthy, beautiful and ne w you!

Conclusion

Thank you again for downloading this book!

I hope this book was able to help you to make delicious foods which will give you a healthy and beautiful skin. Also with the skincare tips, you learnt how you can maintain a vital skin for the rest of your life.

The next step is to try out the recipes and enjoy!

www.ingramcontent.com/pod-product-compliance
Lightning Source LLC
LaVergne TN
LVHW041255150826
845673LV00008B/2600

* 9 7 9 8 4 7 4 1 7 1 4 9 4 *